Ayurveda 101

Ayurveda Basics for
The Absolute Beginner

[Achieve Natural Health and Well Being through Ayurveda]

Advait

Advait

Contents

Advait

Disclaimer and FTC Notice

The intent of the author is only to offer information of a general nature to help you in your quest for emotional, spiritual and physical well being. In the event you use any of the information in this book for yourself, which is your constitutional right, the author and the publisher assume no responsibility for your actions.

Under no circumstances will any legal responsibility or blame be held against the publisher for any reparation, damages, or monetary loss due to the information herein, either directly or indirectly. The information herein is offered for informational purposes solely, and is universal as so. The presentation of the information is without contract or any type of guarantee assurance.

Adherence to all applicable laws and regulations, including international, federal, state, and local governing professional licensing, business practices, advertising, and all other aspects of doing business in the US, Canada, or any other jurisdiction is the sole responsibility of the purchaser or reader.

Neither the author nor the publisher assumes any responsibility or liability whatsoever on the behalf of the purchaser or reader of these materials.

Any perceived slight of any individual or organization is purely unintentional.

Advait

Introduction

Ayurveda (आयुर्वेद) is an ancient system of health care that is native to the Indian subcontinent. It is presently in daily use by millions of people in India and it is been hugely appreciated and followed by millions of people across the globe as a holistic approach to health and well being.

The word 'Ayurveda' is a compound Sanskrit word,

Ayurveda (आयुर्वेद) = Ayushya (आयुष्य) + Veda (वेद),

Where, 'Ayushya' means 'Life' and Veda means 'Wisdom / Knowledge'.

Thus, Ayurveda Literally means, the knowledge of life.

Ayurveda is concerned with measures to protect "Ayushya" (Life), which is achieved through a healthy living along with therapeutic measures that relate to physical, mental, social and spiritual harmony.

Ayurveda has documented cures, for various diseases considered as incurable by modern medical science. Also, most of the modern drugs and medicines are known to have hazardous side-effects while Ayurvedic remedies have none.

People all over the world are now realizing the effectiveness of herbal remedies and are accepting Ayurveda in to their lives.

Advait

Utpatti

Origin of Ayurveda

Mythical origin

According to the mythical accounts, the Ayurveda is attributed to Lord Brahma – The Three Headed Hindu God, regarded as the Creator of the Universe.

Lord Brahma then handed it over to Daksha Prajapati – The Hindu equivalent of Adam.

Daksha Prajapati passed it on to Indra, the King of the Gods.

Indra then taught it to Rishi Bharadwaj, the first of the Maha Yogis.

And, Rishi Bharadwaj passed it on to his disciples who further spread it throughout the Indian sub-continent.

Historical Origin

In the ancient Vedic times, knowledge or information, was never recorded over physical entities, i.e. documentation of information on physical medium like paper (Indian Papyrus called as 'Tamrapatra') was never done.

The teachers used to recite the Veda's and other scripts in front of their disciples and they used to learn it by heart and recall it whenever they required it.

Due to this tradition no one really knows when Ayurveda came into being and the historical origin is the first time when Ayurveda was mentioned in Vedic texts, but Ayurveda is believed to have existed for at least 5000 years before the first mention of it in Vedic texts.

The first historical mention of Ayurveda is attributed to *Maharshi Agnivesh* in his work – *Agnivesh Tantra.* [around 6th Century B.C.]

This works were later redacted and revived by *Maharshi Charaka* and it later became widely known as *Charaka Sanhita.* [1st Century A.D.] (Which formed the basis of Modern Ayurveda.)

The Surgical science under Ayurveda was studied and researched by *Maharshi Dhanvantari* much earlier i.e. around 4th -5th Century B.C.

Maharshi Dhanvantari is regarded and worshipped in India as the God of Medicine and Surgery. His disciple *Sushruta* further created his own work on Ayurveda based on *Dhanvantari's* and his own observations and experiments. His work is widely known as the *'Sushruta Sanhita'* and forms the basis of modern day surgical science.

Ashtaangaveda

The Eight branches of Ayurveda

Ayurveda is further classified in eight different branches which deal with different aspects of medicinal science. They are;

#1 *Kaaya Chikitsa Tantra* – Science of Internal Medicines.

#2 *Shalya Chikitsa* – Science of Surgery.

#3 *Shalakya Tantra* – Branch of Ayurveda which deals with Ears, Nose, Throat & Eyes.

#4 *Kaumaarbhritya Tantra* – Science of Pediatrics.

#5 *Aagada Tantra* – Toxicology

#6 *Vajikarana Tantra* – Science of Genetics.

#7 *Rasaayana Tantra* – Science of Longevity and Health through Food.

#8 *Bhuta Vidya* – Science of Psychiatry and Spiritual Healing.

Advait

Panch Maha Bhuta's

The Five Fundamental Elements

According to Ayurveda, our entire world is made of 'the five fundamental elements' called as *The Panch-Maha-Bhuta's*. The five elements being;

#1 *Prithvi* which means '**Earth**'

#2 *Jal* which means '**Water**'

#3 *Agni* which means '**Fire**'

#4 *Vaayu* which means '**Wind**' and

#5 *Aakash* which means '**Space/Vacuum**'.

They are also called the earth element, water element, fire element, wind element and space element.

These five elements constitute the human body – the nutrients from the soil (earth) are absorbed by the plants which we consume (thus we survive on the earth element), the blood flowing through own veins represents the water element, the body heat represents the fire element, the oxygen we inhale and the carbon dioxide we exhale represents the wind element and the sinuses we have in our nose and skull represent the space element.

Ayurveda 101

As long as these five elements in our body are balanced and maintain appropriate levels we remain healthy. An imbalance of these elements in the human body leads to a deteriorated health and diseases.

The basic principle of Ayurveda is that the entire cosmos or universe is part of one singular absolute.

Everything that exists in the vast external universe (macrocosm) also appears in the internal cosmos of the human body (microcosm). The human body consisting of hundreds of millions of cells, when healthy, is in harmony, self-perpetuating and self-correcting just as the universe is.

In the ancient Ayurvedic text, *Charaka Sanhita*, Mahrshi Charaka says **'Yat Pinde, Tat Bramhande'** which means;

"Man is the epitome of the universe. Within man, there is as much diversity as in the world outside. Similarly, the outside world is as diverse as human beings themselves."

In other words, all human beings are a living microcosm of the universe and the universe is a living macrocosm of human beings.

Advait

Sapta-Dhatu

The Seven Body Tissues

In Ayurveda all the constituents that make up a human body are divided into seven broad categories known as *Sapta-Dhatu's*.

#1 **Rasa Dhatu** – Metabolic Juices and Plasma (The Digestive Syste).

#2 **Rakta Dhatu** – Blood (Circulatory system).

#3 **Mamsa Dhatu** – Muscles and Tendons (Muscular System).

#4 **Med Dhatu** – Bodily Fat.

#5 **Majja Dhatu** – Bone Marrow.

#6 **Asthi Dhatu** – Bones (Skeletal System).

#7 **Shukra Dhatu** – Seminal Fluids (Reproductive System).

Nidaan aevum Chikitsaa

Diagnosis & Treatment

The modern medicinal science basically considers Viruses and Bacteria's as the main cause of any disease, while diagnosis in Ayurveda is based on detailed data obtained from the facts related to a person's habits, physical constitution, psychological constitution, diet, profession etc.

Ayurveda considers the digestive system as the major source of most of the diseases. Any disturbance in the digestive and assimilatory mechanism leads to the formation and accumulation of various types of Toxins (called as *'Ama'*) which cause diseases.

According to Ayurveda any disease intensifies in six stages called as the **'Shada Kriyakaal'** and the first stage begins with digestive disabilities, any disease can be controlled before manifesting if we maintain an efficient and healthy digestive system.

The Essence of Ayurveda lies in Prevention of Disease.

Ayurveda uses three major principles in treating any disease depending upon the stage of the disease. They are:

Advait

#1. *Nidaan Parivarjana* (Prevention)

This involves eradication of the disease producing factors and then imposing preventive measures.

#2. *Shaman Chikitsaa* (Curing)

This involves curative treatment and is applied when the disease is in its early stages.

#3. *Shodhan Chikitsaa* (Purification)

This involves purification techniques and is applied when the disease is advanced and has affected the dhatus.

Along with curing the disease, Ayurveda rejuvenates the body of an individual and also increases his/her immunity against the disease producing organism. The Ayurvedic treatments act as a tonic and tone-up our bodily systems.

The Three Dosha's and Your Prakriti

Vata – Pitta – Kapha

The core concept of Ayurvedic medicine is that, the five fundamental elements integrate into physical form as the three *Doshas* and health exists when there is a balance between the three fundamental bodily *Doshas* known as: *Vata, Pitta* and *Kapha.*

The Dosha – Element Relationship

Vata Dosha – Air Element + Space/vacuum Element

Pitta Dosha – Fire Element + Water Element

Kapha Dosha – Water Element + Earth Element

The physical volume of a human being is mainly composed of *Kapha,* the chemical processes and reactions taking place in the body are due to the manifestation of *Pitta*, and the bodily movements and activities are attributed to *Vata.*

For an individual to remain healthy, these three basic substances (*doshas*) must be in equilibrium. Any kind

Advait

of disequilibrium of these *doshas* will cause disintegration of the body which leads to disease.

When we consume food, it is digested and nutrients (*Saara*) and waste/excreta (*Mala*) are produced. The nutrients nourish the seven bodily tissues (*SaptaDhatu's*) and the waste is thrown out of the body through sweat, urine, feces, nasal discharge, eye discharge etc., while this is happening the three doshas move from one part of the body to another part and induce sound health, resistance to disease and physical strength in an individual. But, if the *doshas* are excited or vitiated they produce disease in the body.

Vata

Vata is the air principle necessary to mobilize the function of the nervous system.

The main functions of *Vata* are to give motion to the body, conduction of impulses from sensory organs, separation of nutrient and waste from food, secretion of urine and semen.

In healthy condition it performs all the physiological functions in the body, it is responsible for speech & hearing, it regulates the normal circulation in the body and it is also responsible for formation and development of foetus in intra-uterine stage.

When excited or vitiated, it produces psychosomatic disorder, causes weight loss, loss of physical strength and it may cause congenital deformities.

Types and Location of Vata

Based upon the function and effective location, *Vata* is of five types:

#1 Praan Vata

#2 Udaan Vata

#3 Vyaan Vata

#4 Apaan Vata

Advait

The *Praan Vata* is located in the upper chest cavity, tongue, nose and head. Its most important function is mind control and respiration.

The *Udaan Vata* is located in the umbilical region and neck. It is responsible for nasal functions.

The *Vyaan Vata* mainly resides in the chest cavity around the heart and travels all around the body. It is responsible for blood circulation throughout the body and also for other bodily movements.

The *Apaan Vata* is located in intestine, rectum and urinary bladder. Its main function is evacuation of urine, secretion of semen and expulsion of feces.

The *Samaan Vata* is located in the stomach and is responsible for digestion of the food and separation of waste from nutrients. It also regulates the temperature of the body and one of its most important functions is to influence the movement of *Pitta* and *Kapha*.

Pitta

Pitta is the fire principle which uses bile to direct digestion and hence metabolism into the venous system.

The endocrine functions in the body and other biological activities in the human body are caused by *Pitta*. It is the by-product of human blood (Rakta).

Pitta is homologous of blood and both are situated/originate in spleen and liver.

Pitta can be physically observed, it is a yellow coloured viscous liquid, it has a fleshy and unpleasant smell and it feels hot when touched.

Pitta provides volume and colour to blood, induces proper digestion, proper vision. It is responsible for body heat, appetite, thirst, complexion and intelligence.

Types and Location of Pitta

Based upon the function and effective location, *Pitta* is of five types:

#1 Paachak Pitta

#2 Ranjak Pitta

#3 Saadhak Pitta

Advait

#4 Alochak Pitta

#5 Bhraajak Pitta

The *Paachak Pitta* is located between the stomach and duodenum, when excited/aggravated it causes a burning sensation, increases appetite, thirst, causes yellowness of urine, feces and eyes.

The *Ranjak Pitta* is located in the liver and spleen and its essential function is to induce the formation of blood in liver and spleen.

The *Saadhak Pitta* is located in the chest cavity around the heart and is mainly responsible for intelligence and enthusiasm.

The *Alochak Pitta* is located around the eye sockets and it helps in vision.

The *Bhraajak Pitta* is located in the skin all around the body. It maintains the health of the skin and regulates the body temperature.

Kapha

Kapha is the water principle which relates to mucous, lubrication and the carrier of nutrients into the arterial system.

When compared to *Vata* and *Pitta*, *Kapha* is the most stable of the three doshas and it is mainly composed of water. It is responsible for formation of bodily structures.

It is white in colour, thick, viscous, slimy and soft to touch. The body owes its softness, smoothness, moisture and coolness to *Kapha*.

The *Kapha* joints together various structures of the body and the joints. It promotes healing, immunity and tissue-building within the body. *Kapha* provides stability, physical strength and sturdiness to one's body.

Types and Location of Kapha

Based upon the function and effective location, *Kapha* is of five types:

#1 Kledak Kapha

#2 Avalambak Kapha

#3 Bodhak Kapha

Advait

#4 Tarpak Kapha

#5 Sleshmak Kapha

The *Kledak Kapha* is located in the stomach and its primary function is to moisten the food material and aiding digestion.

The *Avalambak Kapha* is located in and around the heart and its primary function is to nourish, protect and lubricate the heart.

The *Bodhak Kapha* is located at the back (root) of the tongue and in the pharynx and it is responsible for the *perception* of taste.

The *Tarpak Kapha* is located in the head/skull cavity and its main function is to nourish the brain and to maintain the sensory functions.

The *Sleshmak Kapha* is located in our joints. It is oily and viscous in nature and it nourishes the joints and keeps them lubricated.

Prakriti *(The Basic Bodily Constitution)*

According to Ayurveda, every person is constituted of the Three Dosha's - The *Vata* Dosha, The *Pitta* Dosha and The *Kapha* Dosha.

And, any one of the three Dosha's is most dominant among them, which determines the basic or primary constitution or *Prakriti* of an individual. For example, a person with a dominant *Pitta* Dosha is said to have a '*Pitta Prakriti*' as his primary *Prakriti*.

Ayurveda is all about appeasing the dominant Dosha and maintaining a good balance between the other two Dosha's.

Want to know if you have a *Vata, Pitta* or *Kapha* Prakriti?? Then turn the page and take the test.

Advait

The three doshas test for determining your Prakriti

In this test you will be asked a series of questions, with three options available to choose from as your answer.

At the end of the test,

If the majority of your answers is **'A'** then your primary Prakriti is *Vata Prakriti.*

If the majority of your answers is **'B'** then your primary Prakriti is *Pitta Prakriti.*

If the majority of your answers is **'C'** then your primary Prakriti is *Kapha Prakriti.*

Here's the Test.

#1 Your Frame

A.   Thin, Lanky, boney and taller or shorter than average.

B.   Average build and size with weight centered in middle.

C.   Heavy, Stocky, Broad and either very tall or very short.

#2 Your Weight

A.   Low with difficulties in gaining weight.

B.   Moderate, no difficulties in gaining or losing weight.

C.   Heavy with difficulties in gaining weight.

#3 Your Appetite

A.   Unpredictable and irregular.

B.   Strong, you cannot skip meals and need to eat after every 3-4 hrs.

C.   Constant but can skip meals easily and tolerate hunger.

#4 Amount of food you eat

A.   Variable, sometimes a lot and sometimes very little.

B.   More, you can eat large quantities at once.

C.   Comparatively less.

#5 The Weather you Prefer

A.   Warm climates and dislike windy dry and cold days.

B.   Cooler climates and dislike heat.

C.   A lot adaptable to climate but absolutely dislike cold and rainy days.

#6 Your Skin Texture

A.   Thin and dry but rough and cool to touch.

B.   Smooth and Warm with an Oily T-zone.

C.   Thick and Greasy and cold to touch.

Advait

#7 How do you Walk?

A.   Fast with light steps.

B.   Determined steps at an average speed.

C.   Steady steps at a slow pace.

#8 Your Complexion

A.   Dark and tans easily.

B.   Fair with freckles and prone to sunburn.

C.   Pale and difficult to tan.

#9 The way you sleep

A.   A light sleeper and gets awakened very easily.

B.   Sleeps deep and even, hardly needs more than 8 hrs of sleep.

C.   Long and sound sleeper, have difficulty in waking up after a long sleep.

#10 Your Hair

A.   Dry, brittle and curly.

B.   Soft and Straight.

C.   Thick and Wavy, tends to become greasy.

Advait

#11 Your Perspiration

A.   Very little with little odor.

B.   Intense when it gets hot, and has a sharp smell.

C.   Constant and moderate with a sweet smell.

#12 Your Eyes

A.   Small and dry, you blink a lot.

B.   Penetrating gaze, reddish sclerae.

C.   Large and moist with a white sclerae.

#13 Your Body Temperature

A.   Less than normal, with cold feet and hands.

B.   More than normal, with palms, feet and face warm or hot.

C.   Normal but palms and feet are cold.

#14 Your Lips

A.   Thin and dry and are often chapped.

B.   Pink and Soft.

C.   Full and Smooth.

Advait

#15 Your Voice

A.   Low volume, hoarse and cracking.

B.   Loud and Sharp.

C.   Pleasant and Harmonious with a low pitch.

#16 Your Teeth

A.   Crooked and irregular with receding gums.

B.   Yellowish with easily bleeding gums.

C.   Large, white and straight.

#17. Your Fingers and Nails

A.   Delicate, small and long fingers with chipped nails.

B.   Regular fingers with pink and soft nails.

C.   Wide and angular fingers with large and hard nails.

Advait

Vata Lakshana

Vata Personal Traits

People with a *Vata* constitution aren't usually physically well developed and have poor muscle development. They are either tall or short and have scanty hairs. Their eyes lack a healthy watery glean and are usually small and dry.

They don't usually have a strong digestive system and they love sweet and sour foods.

The *Mala* (Excreta) tendency of these people is less, i.e. they perspire less, they urinate less and the feces is usually scanty and dry.

On an intellectual level, they have a very good understanding of things but they struggle with sharp memory and tend to forget a lot.

Ideal Diet for a person with *Vata* Prakriti

Fruits you should eat:

Sweet Fruits, Apricots, Avocado, Bananas, Berries, Cherries, Coconut, Figs(fresh), Grapefruit, Grapes, Lemons, Mango, Melons (sweet), Oranges, Papaya, Peaches, Pineapples, Plums.

Fruits you should avoid:

Dried Fruits, Apples, Cranberries, Pears, Persimmon, Pomegranate, Watermelon.

Vegetables you should eat:

Cooked Vegetables, Asparagus, Beets, Carrots, Cucumber, Garlic, Green Beans, Okra (cooked), Onion (cooked), Potato (sweet), Radishes, Zucchini.

Vegetables you should avoid:

Raw Vegetables, Broccoli, Brussels, Sprouts, Cabbage, Cauliflower, Celery, Eggplant, Mushrooms, Onions (raw), Peas, Peppers.

Advait

Grains you should eat:

Rice, Wheat, Oats (cooked).

Grains you should avoid:

Barley, Buckwheat, Corn, Millet, Rye.

Pitta Lakshana

Pitta Personal Traits

People with a *Pitta* constitution are moderately developed with slender bodies. They are broad chested and their muscles are adequately developed.

They have a medium height and possess thin, silky hair. Their eye's are always moist and are usually grey in colour.

They have a strong digestive system, thus inducing a healthy appetite. They like sweet a lot.

The *Mala* (Excreta) tendency of these people is high, i.e. they perspire a lot, they urinate a lot (large volume) and the feces is moist and high in volume.

Intellectually they are sharp and possess good comprehensive and oratory skills.

Advait

Ideal Diet for a person with *Pitta* Prakriti

Fruits you should eat:

Sweet Fruits, Apples, Avocado, Coconut, Figs, Grapes (dark), Mango, Oranges (sweet), Pears, Pineapples (sweet), Plums (sweet), Pomegranate, Prunes, Raisins.

Fruits you should avoid:

Sour Fruits, Apricots, Berries, Bananas, Cherries, Cranberries, Grapefruit, Grapes (green), Lemons, Oranges (sour), Papaya, Peaches.

Vegetables you should eat:

Sweet & Bitter Vegetables, Asparagus, Broccoli, Brussels Sprouts, Cabbage, Cucumber, Cauliflower, Celery, Green Beans, Leafy Greens, Lettuce, Mushrooms, Okra, Peas, Parsley, Peppers (green), Potatoes, Sprouts, Zucchini.

Vegetables you should avoid:

Pungent Vegetables, Beets, Carrots, Eggplant, Peppers (hot), Radishes, Spinach, Tomatoes.

Grains you should eat:

Barley, Oats (cooked), Rice, Wheat.

Grains you should avoid:

Buckwheat, Corn, Millet, Oats (dry), Rye.

Advait

Kapha Lakshana

Kapha Personal Traits

People with a *Kapha* constitution have well developed bodies but tend to be a bit over-weight. They have highly developed muscles and have a broad chest.

They tend to be tall and have thick, wavy hair. They possess attractive black or blue eyes.

Though they have a slow digestive system, they have a moderate and regular appetite, and they like pungent and bitter food.

The *Mala* (Excreta) tendency of these people is moderate, i.e. they perspire and urinate in moderate quantities and their feces are moist and moderate in volume.

They are usually calm and loving people with a very good and sharp memory. They find it a bit difficult to understand new things, but once understood they never forget.

Ideal Diet for a person with *Kapha* Prakriti

Fruits you should eat:

Apples, Apricots, Berries, Cherries, Cranberries, Figs (dry), Mango, Peaches, Pears, Persimmon, Pomegranate, Prunes, Raisins.

Fruits you should avoid:

Sweet & Sour Fruits, Avocado, Bananas, Coconut, Figs (fresh), Grapefruit, Grapes, Lemons, Melons, Oranges, Papaya, Pineapples, Plums.

Vegetables you should eat:

Pungent & Bitter Vegetables, Asparagus, Beets, Broccoli, Brussels Sprouts, Cabbage, Cauliflower, Celery, Eggplant, Garlic, Leafy Greens, Lettuce, Mushrooms, Okra, Onions, Parsley, Peas, Peppers.

Vegetables you should avoid:

Sweet & Juicy Vegetables, Cucumber, Potatoes (sweet), Tomatoes, Zucchini.

Advait

Grains you should eat:

Barley, Corn, Millet, Oats (dry), Rice (Basmati, small amount), Rye.

Grains you should avoid:

Oats (cooked), Rice (brown), Rice (white), Wheat.

Jathar Agni

Digestive Fire

Agni is the Sanskrit word for 'Fire' and Ayurveda regards Digestion as a holy fire which produces energy for sustaining life.

The Digestive Fire or *Jathar-Agni* is of key importance in Ayurveda.

Ayurveda mentions four types of *Jathar-Agni's*;

#1 **Sama Agni** – Balanced, proper digestion with no after effects.

#2 **Vishama Agni** – Irregular Digestion with formation of gases and bloating as after effects.

#3 **Tikshna Agni** – Sharp Digestion with acid reflux and heartburn as after effects.

#4 **Manda Agni** – Slow Digestion inducing dullness and laziness.

Advait

When your *Jathar-Agni* is not functioning at an optimal level *(Sama Agni)*, **Ama** (the toxic by-product of undigested food) clogs the channels. In due time, this clogging forms the root cause for diseases, hence Ayurveda, has given a paramount importance to keep your Digestive Fire strong and balanced if you wish to lead a healthy life throughout your life.

Trayodasha Vega

13 Natural Urge's

Vega is the Sanskrit word for 'Natural Urge'.

Ayurveda considers our body as a self-rectifying microcosm, and it defines the 'Natural Urges' or Vega's as our bodies attempt for self-healing and for achieving a healthy equilibrium.

Ayurveda mentions *13 Natural Urges*, which should never be suppressed, since suppressing them can cause serious physical and psychological disorders.

The 13 natural Urges which **should not be suppressed** are;

#1 Crying

#2 Yawning

#3 Hunger

#4 Thirst

#5 Sleep

#6 Breath

#7 Urination

#8 Defecation

Advait

Rogpratirodhan

The Preventive Measures

Prevention is of disease in of paramount importance in the Ayurvedic medicinal system. The prescribed preventive measures can be classified into five categories:

#1 *Swasthavritti* (hygiene)

It involves inculcating routine, hygienic habits like brushing teeth, taking a bath, regular exercise, Shatapavali *(walking at least 100 steps after a meal)*, rising up early etc.

#2 *Ritucharya* (Seasonal Routine)

It involves specific regimens and diets that are to be followed in various seasons.

#3 *Sadvritti (Good Nature)*

It involves recommendations for a decent social behavior which contributes towards psychological well being.

Advait

#4 Yogachar (Practise of Yoga)

It involves regular practice of various *Yoga Asana's* and *Pranayaam*.

#5 Rasaayan Tantra (Use of Herbal Potions)

It involves regular use of rejuvenating and virile herbal potions which act as tonic for the body.

Chikitsatantra

Curative Measures

The curative measures mentioned in Ayurveda are three-fold:

Internal Medicine

External Medicine

Surgery

Internal Medicine

Internal medicine is a major discipline in the practice of Ayurveda.

Preparation recipes of thousands of drugs are found in Ayurveda. These medicines are made from herbs, minerals and even biological products. The most commonly used internal medicines are;

Klitaka (Paste)

It is prepared by grinding fresh herbs on mortar with a pestle.

Advait

Swaras (Strained Juice)

It is prepared by forming a paste first and then straining the paste through a thin cloth (by applying pressure) to obtain the juice of the herbs.

Churna (powder)

It is prepared by grinding dried herbs.

Ugal (Infusion)

It is prepared by adding one(1) part of Churna (powder) to eight(8) parts of hot water, keep it unstirred for some time and then strained through a cloth. (Similar to preparing *tea*)

Kaadha (Decoction)

It is prepared by boiling one(1) part of herbal paste with sixteen(16) parts of water and reducing the mixture to 1/4th .

External Medicine

As the name suggests, it is the external application of medicinal preparations. The preparations that are applied externally are pastes, powders, powders

Ayurveda 101

converted to pastes by adding water, bathing solutions prepared by adding medicinal infusions to the bath water, gargling using infusions etc.

Surgery

Ayurveda was the first medicinal system in the world to perform different type of operations (*shalyachikitsaa*), sewing up wounds, treating fractures by operating procedures and Ayurveda even has historical accounts of damaged/burnt skin patches being replaced by healthy skin patches (*Plastic Surgery*).

Conclusion

Ayurveda is the oldest medicinal science which originated in the ancient Vedic culture and many of the western healing techniques have their roots in Ayurveda hence, it is called 'Mother of All healing'.

The core concept of Ayurveda which is given utmost importance is *Rogpratirodha* i.e. prevention of disease through hygienic habits, appropriate diet, regular exercise (yoga), right thinking and use of various herbs as tonics.

Knowing Ayurveda enables an individual to maintain a perfect equilibrium of body, mind & soul thus achieving everlasting health and happiness.

~~~

Excerpt

Super Herbs: 25 Ultimate Ayurvedic Herbs with Magical Healing Powers and How To Use Them

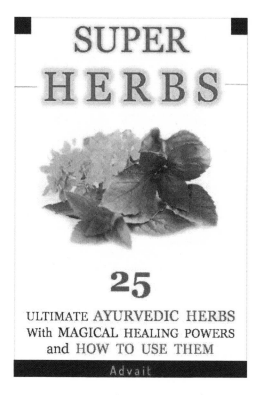

Turn the Page →

Advait

Important

In modern botanical terms, a herb is considered as a plant with a non-woody stem, which has a very short lifespan and which withers away after flowering.

In Ayurveda, a herb is called as *Aushadhi Vanaspati* ('औषधी वनस्पति') i.e. a plant whose leaves, stems, roots, flowers, fruits or seeds have medicinal uses. This criterion is the basis of the 25 herbs included in this book.

Let's get started...

Herb #1

Cardamom

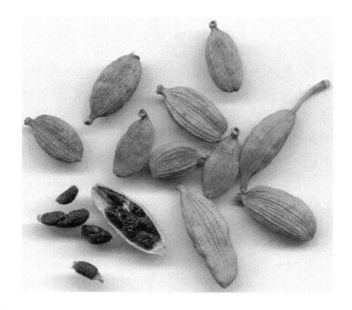

Ayurvedic Name: *Elaichi*

Botanical Name: *Ellettaria Cardamomum*

Origin & Physical Properties:

Advait

In India Cardamom is called as the 'Queen of Spices' and rightly so is one of the most valued spices in the world.

Cardamom grows as a perennial herb with very large leaves and white or pale green flowers.

The dried cardamom fruits of the plant have healing properties.

Originating in Southern India this spice moved westwards and was extensively used for consumption and as medicine. The earliest mention of cardamom in the western world is by *Theophrastus* in 4th Century B.C.

Healing Properties:

The aroma and the healing properties of the cardamom are owing to the volatile oil in its seeds. It is mainly used for relieving flatulence and for strengthening the digestive system.

In Digestive Disorders

Cardamom rectifies air element and water element imbalance in the body. It is helpful in relieving gas and heart-burn.

* Ground Cardamom seeds mixed with Ginger, Cloves and Coriander, is an effective remedy for indigestion.

In Bad Breath

Cardamom is an extremely effective mouth freshener. Chewing a few seeds will cure bad breath.

In Genital & Urinary Disorders

* Powdered cardamom seeds mixed with a tablespoon of banana leaf and *Amla(Indian Gooseberry)* juice should be consumed for treating gonorrhea, cystitis, scanty urination or to cure burning sensation during urination.

In Depression

* Powdered cardamom seeds when added while brewing tea gives it a pleasant aroma and is a very common remedy for treating depression.

In Impotency

Cardamom works like a charm in treatment of sexual dysfunction and premature ejaculation.

* A pinch of cardamom seed powder boiled in milk and sweetened with honey when taken every night yields excellent results.

Advait

**Very Important

It is specified throughout Ayurveda, that *'excessive use of anything should be avoided; any good thing which is a life saver in small quantities is poisonous if taken in large quantities over a long period of time'*.

Herb #2

Clove

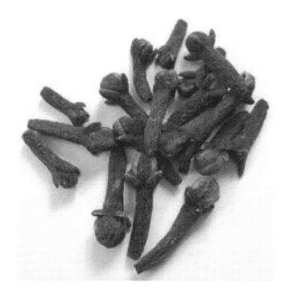

Ayurvedic Name: *Laung / Lavang*

Botanical Name: *Syzygium aromaticum*

Origin & Physical Properties:

Advait

Clove is the dried unopened flower bud obtained from an evergreen tree growing up to 12 meters.

Clove is being extensively used in India for the past 3,000 years.

Historical references show cloves being imported in Alexandria in 176 A.D.

Healing Properties:

Clove has stimulating properties; it helps in regulating blood circulation and in relieving flatulence.

In Digestive Disorders

Cloves are extremely useful in cases of gastric irritability and dyspepsia.

* Powder of fired cloves when mixed with a spoon of honey and consumed is very effective in controlling vomiting.

Cough

Chewing a clove with a crystal on common salt eases expectoration and soothes the throat.

* 3-4 drops of clove oil + Spoonful of honey + a clove of garlic, help in soothing spasmodic coughs in Asthma and Bronchitis. (should be taken before sleeping)

Ayurveda 101

Asthma

Clove is a very effective remedy for asthma.

* Boil 5-6 cloves in a cup of water, add a spoonful of honey. Consume thrice daily.

In Bad Breath & Toothache

Clove is an extremely effective mouth freshener. Chewing a single clove will cure bad breath and clove oil when applied to a tooth cavity in a decayed tooth relieves toothache.

In Muscular Cramping

Muscular cramping is immediately relieved by applying clove oil to the affected area.

Advait

Herb #3

Dandelion

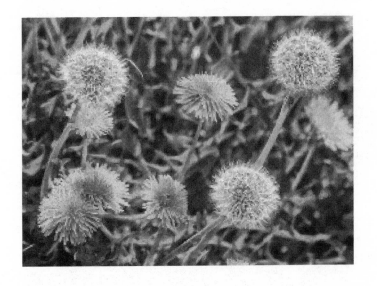

Ayurvedic Name: *Kaanphool*

Botanical Name: *Taraxacum officinale*

Origin & Physical Properties:

Dandelion is a perennial herb which is extensively used as a tasty salad vegetable.

Dandelion is native to Europe. It is a very common plant and grows wild almost everywhere.

Nutritionally, you will be surprised to know that it contains as much Iron as Spinach and 4 times more vitamin A than Lettuce.

Healing Properties:

In Bone Disorders

The juice obtained from the leaves and stem of Dandelion is mixed with juices of the leaves of carrots and turnips for curing bone disorders.

In Liver and Gall Bladder Disorders

Regular consumption of Dandelion benefits our Liver and Gall Bladder which are essential organs for handling fats within the body and for detoxification.

* A Hepatitis patient can greatly benefit from drinking Dandelion Tea, which is a brew made of boiling dandelion roots.

In Urinary Disorders

Advait

Dandelion when consumed increases the quantity and flow of Urine and cures any other urinary tract disorders.

Dandelion Coffee

Dandelion Coffee is made from its dried, roasted and ground roots. It's a natural and organic beverage without any harmful effects of regular coffee.

Herb #4

Garlic

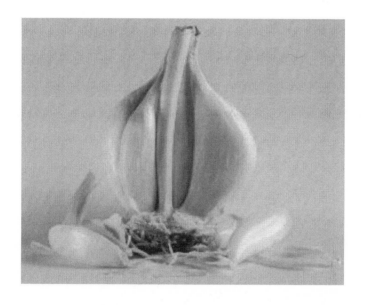

Ayurvedic Name: *Lahsoon*

Botanical Name: *Allium Sativum*

Origin & Physical Properties:

Advait

Garlic is a biennial herb of the onion family. It has a flattened stem and narrow, flat leaves.

Garlic originated in Central Asia and still remains one of the staple spices of various Asian cuisines.

*** Do You Know*

Garlic was a part of the monthly salary of the Pyramid builders of ancient Egypt. They even went on a strike when Garlic was not provided to them and resumed work only after Garlic was reinstated as a part of their salaries.

Healing Properties:

In Ayurveda, Garlic has been used for treating cough, asthma, leprosy, arteriosclerosis, fever, worms and a lot of other disorders.

In Digestive Disorders

Garlic is one of the most beneficial herbs for the digestive system. It stimulates the movement of intestines and aids in secretion of digestive juices.

It has an antiseptic effect and is an excellent remedy for infectious diseases and inflammations of the stomach and intestine.

Garlic is also an excellent worm expeller.

In High Blood Pressure

Garlic is one of the most effective remedy for lowering blood pressure. It also works like a charm in curing arrhythmia.

In Arteriosclerosis

When consumed regularly garlic prevents arteriosclerosis.

In Blood Disorders

Garlic is the best natural rejuvenator. It removes toxins from the blood, revitalizes the body and stimulates circulation.

It is the only food ingredient known to man, which when consumed promotes and fertilizes essential intestinal flora while at the same time killing the harmful bacteria, truly a miracle herb.

Advait

Herb #5

Nutmeg

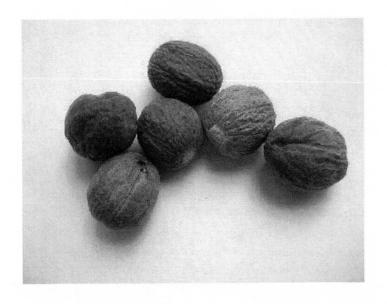

Ayurvedic Name: *Jaiphal*

Botanical Name: *Myristica fragrans*

Origin & Physical Properties:

Ayurveda 101

Nutmeg is the dried kernel of the seeds of the Nutmeg tree.

It has a strong aroma with a slightly bitter taste.

Nutmeg trees originated in Asia and are now abundant in Indonesia, Malaysia and Sri Lanka.

Healing Properties:

Nutmeg is used in the preparation of various Ayurvedic medicines since ancient times. The oil extracted from it is used in liniments, perfumery and as an antispasmodic.

In Digestive Disorders

* Nutmeg powder (about 4-5 grams) taken with a tablespoon of *Amla*(Indian Gooseberry) 3 to 4 times a day is effective for indigestion and morning sickness.

In Insomnia

Nutmeg powder mixed with *Amla* juice is also an effective medicine for insomnia.

* A pinch of Nutmeg powder mixed with a few drops of honey, is given to infants who cry at night, to induce sleep. (Do not follow this method regularly and take your doctor's advice before doing it.)

Advait

As a Sex Stimulant

* A pinch of Nutmeg powder mixed with a tablespoon of Honey and a half-boiled egg, when consumed an hour before sex acts as an excellent stimulant and also prolongs the duration of sexual act.

In Skin Disorders

Nutmeg is very effective in treatment of skin diseases like ringworm and eczema.

Want to read further??...

Get it here,
https://www.amazon.com/dp/B00QCYGQBA

Thank You

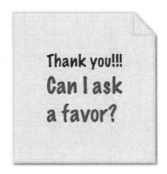

Thank you so much for reading my book. I hope you really liked it.

As you probably know, many people look at the reviews on Amazon before they decide to purchase a book.

If you liked the book, please take a minute to leave a review with your feedback.

60 seconds is all I'm asking for, and it would mean a lot to me.

Thank You so much.

All the best,

Advait

Advait

Other Books by Advait

On Ayurvedic Healing

Ayurveda of Diet: 15 Ultimate Eating Habits
Recommended in Ayurveda for Health and Healing

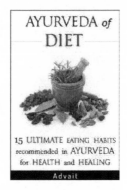

http://www.amazon.com/dp/BooNKPDCUW

<u>My Other Books</u>
<u>On Mudras</u>

Mudras for Awakening Chakras: 19 Simple Hand
Gestures for Awakening & Balancing Your Chakras

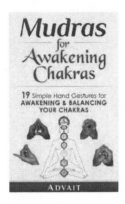

http://www.amazon.com/dp/B00P82COAY

[#1 Bestseller in 'Yoga']

[#1 Bestseller in 'Chakras']

Advait

Mudras for Weight Loss: 21 Simple Hand Gestures for Effortless Weight Loss

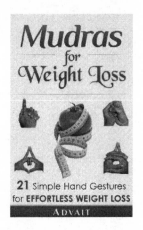

http://www.amazon.com/dp/B00P3ZPSEK

Mudras for Spiritual Healing: 21 Simple Hand
Gestures for Ultimate Spiritual Healing & Awakening

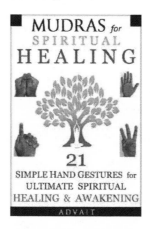

http://www.amazon.com/dp/B00PFYZLQO

Advait

Mudras for Sex: 25 Simple Hand Gestures for
Extreme Erotic Pleasure & Sexual Vitality

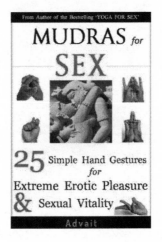

http://www.amazon.com/dp/B00OJR1DRY

Ayurveda 101

Mudras: 25 Ultimate techniques for Self Healing

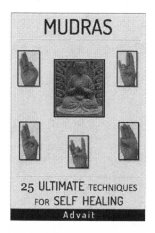

http://www.amazon.com/dp/B00MMPB5CI

Advait

Mudras for a Strong Heart: 21 Simple Hand Gestures
for Preventing, Curing & Reversing Heart Disease

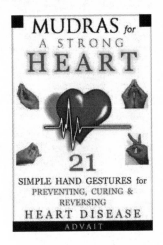

http://www.amazon.com/dp/BooPFRLGTM

Ayurveda 101

Mudras for Anxiety: 25 Simple Hand Gestures for Curing Your Anxiety

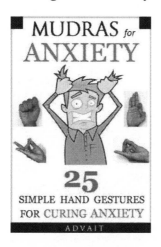

http://www.amazon.com/dp/B00PF011IU

Advait

Mudras for Memory Improvement: 25 Simple Hand Gestures for Ultimate Memory Improvement

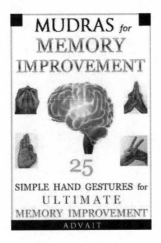

http://www.amazon.com/dp/B00PFSP8TK

Mudras for Stress Management: 21 Simple Hand
Gestures for a Stress Free Life

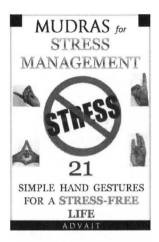

http://amazon.com/dp/B00PFTJ6OC

Advait

Mudras for Curing Cancer: 21 Simple Hand Gestures
for Preventing & Curing Cancer

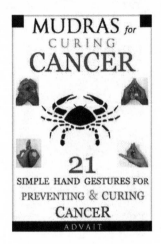

http://www.amazon.com/dp/B00PFO199M

Ayurveda 101

On Yoga

Easy Yoga: Your Ultimate Beginners Guide to Understanding Yoga and Leading a Disease-Free Life through Routine Yoga Practice

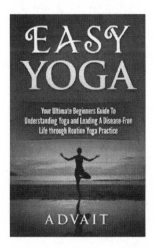

http://www.amazon.com/dp/B010I97366

Advait

Monday Yoga: Pranayam and Sukshma-Asana's for starting Your Routine Yoga Practice and Inducing Vigor into Your Life on the first day of the Week

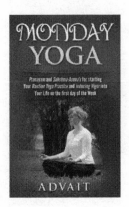

http://www.amazon.com/dp/B011SI6MK4

(This book is available for FREE)

Tuesday Yoga: 12 Yoga Asanas to be performed on
Tuesday as a Part of Your Daily Yoga Routine

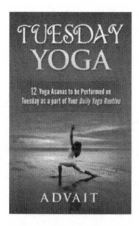

http://www.amazon.com/dp/B013GGA1AS

Advait

Wednesday Yoga: 12 Yoga Asanas to be performed on
Wednesday as a Part of Your Daily Yoga Routine

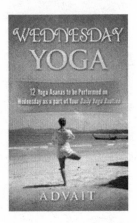

http://www.amazon.com/dp/B014RTDQ5U

Ayurveda 101

Thursday Yoga: 12 Yoga Asanas to be performed on
Thursday as a Part of Your Daily Yoga Routine

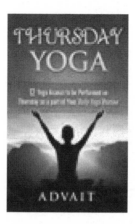

http://www.amazon.com/dp/B015JMSEPQ

Advait

Friday Yoga: 12 Yoga Asanas to be performed on
Friday as a Part of Your Daily Yoga Routine

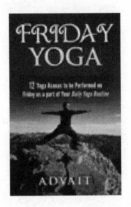

http://www.amazon.com/dp/B015UK17KG

Saturday Yoga: 12 Yoga Asanas to be Performed on
Saturday as a Part of Your Daily Yoga Routine

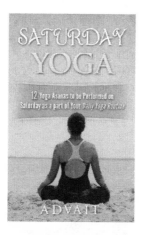

http://www.amazon.com/dp/B0165WFUJW

Advait

Sunday Yoga: Suryanamaskar (Sun Salutation) & 5
Yoga Asanas for a Blissful Culmination of Your Daily
Yoga Routine

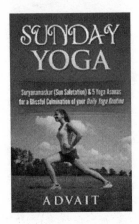

http://www.amazon.com/dp/B016Q8GF8K

Advait

Ayurveda 101

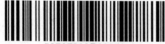

Made in the USA
Lexington, KY
14 January 2017